GALLBLADDER SURGERY RECOVERY DIET

Comprehensive Guide Unlocking The Secrets of nutrition after Surgery Success, Nourishing Meal Plans, Recipes And Practical Tips For Optimal Health And Wellness)

DR. ALLAN FREDA

Contents

1. Understanding Gallbladder Surgery: This part gives an overview of gallbladder surgery, including why it is done, any possible side effects, and how important it is to change your diet after surgery.

2. The Healing Diet: Look at several healing foods that are designed to help you get better after surgery.

These foods are made to be easy on the digestive system while still giving you the nutrients you need to heal properly.

3. food Plans: Find food plans that can be changed to fit your specific dietary needs and tastes while you're recovering.

These plans know how important it is to eat a variety of foods and tell you how much to eat and when to eat it.

4. Expert Tips for Long-Term Wellness: Get tips from experts on how to live a healthy life after you're better.

To keep your digestive system healthy, learn what foods to eat, how to deal with symptoms, and how to avoid future problems linked to gallbladder health.

Copyright © 2024 Allan Freda.

Disclaimer

The information in this book is for informational purposes only and should not replace professional medical advice, diagnosis, or treatment. Always consult your physician or a qualified health provider regarding any medical concerns. Do not disregard professional medical advice or delay seeking it based on information in this book.

The author does not endorse or have affiliations with any mentioned entities. References are for informational purposes only.

Consult your healthcare provider before making dietary or lifestyle changes, especially during recovery from surgery, as individual needs vary.

Results may vary, and the information provided is not guaranteed to produce specific outcomes.

By reading this book, you acknowledge and agree to consult your healthcare provider before implementing any information herein.

For further guidance, consult your healthcare provider or reputable medical websites for reliable information on surgery recovery diets.

CHAPTER 1

HOW TO GET BETTER AFTER GALLBLADDER SURGERY

Getting Started with Gallbladder Surgery:

Getting rid of the gallbladder is often done through gallbladder surgery, which is also called cholecystectomy. The gallbladder is a small organ that sits under the liver and stores bile, which is a digestive fluid that the liver makes. Gallstones are hard deposits that can stop the flow of bile and cause pain, inflammation, and other problems. They are the most common reason for gallbladder surgery. Depending on the person's health and medical history, gallbladder surgery can be either open surgery or slightly invasive laparoscopic surgery.

Why diet is important for recovery:

What you eat is very important for getting better after gallbladder surgery.

Getting rid of the gallbladder can change how the body breaks down and uses fats, which can change what you need to eat. Following the right food after surgery can help reduce pain, speed up recovery, and avoid problems like digestive problems and lack of nutrients. A well-planned diet can also help with long-term health and wellness, making sure that people can keep up a healthy, balanced eating routine after surgery.

Advice on what to eat after surgery:

It's important to follow certain dietary rules after gallbladder surgery to help the body heal and reduce pain. One of the most important things to think about is slowly adding foods back into the diet so that the body can get used to the new bile flow and digestion. At first, a clear liquid meal may be suggested to keep the digestive system from working too hard and to lower the risk of feeling sick and throwing up. Some of these are gelatine, clear fruit drinks, and broth. People can move on to a full liquid diet, which includes smooth soups, yogurt, and protein shakes, as their tolerance grows.

In the weeks after gallbladder surgery, a low-fat diet is usually suggested as long as it is safe to follow. This means staying away from fatty and high-fat foods that might be hard to digest, like fried foods, fatty meats, and sweets that are high in sugar and fat. Instead, eat more whole grains, fruits, veggies, lean protein sources, and less fat.

Fiber-rich foods can help keep digestion in check and keep you from getting constipated, which can happen after surgery. Getting plenty of water throughout the day is also important to stay fresh.

People can slowly start eating healthy fats again as their healing goes on. Olive oil, nuts, avocados, and other healthy fats are all good examples. However, it's important to keep an eye on tolerance and make changes to the diet as needed to avoid pain or stomach problems. Some people may find that certain foods make their symptoms worse, like bloating, gas, or diarrhea, and may need to avoid or eat less of these foods.

Besides what you eat, it's important to live a good life in general, which includes getting enough rest and regular exercise. This can help your body heal and make you feel better overall while you're recovering from gallbladder surgery. Talking to a doctor or qualified dietitian can help you get the personalised advice and support you need to make the most of your diet after surgery.

Problems that often come up during recovery:

Recovery from gallbladder surgery can be hard for some people in many ways, including with their food and their bodies. One typical problem is getting used to changes in digestion and bowel habits that can happen after the gallbladder is removed or when the flow of bile changes.

As the body gets used to these changes, some people may have diarrhea, bloating, or stomach pain.

A diet low in fat and high in fiber can help keep digestion in check and lessen these effects over time.

Managing food preferences and limits can be hard while you're recovering, especially when you need to stay away from high-fat or greasy foods that may make your symptoms worse. Going to social events or eating out while following a certain diet plan can be hard, but planning and talking to others can help people make smart decisions and stay on track with their healing goals.

Also, some people may have emotional or mental problems while they are recovering, like anxiety, sadness, or anger over having to change their eating habits or deal with physical limitations.

To deal with these worries and keep a positive outlook on recovery, it's important to put yourself first and get help from healthcare professionals, family members, or support groups as required.

Overall, getting better after gallbladder surgery takes time, patience, and being proactive about making changes to your food and way of life. Following post-surgery dietary rules, dealing with common problems, and putting self-care first can help people heal, feel less pain, and be healthy and active for a long time after surgery.

CHAPTER 2
WHAT YOU NEED FOR A HEALING DIET

A carefully planned post-surgery diet is necessary to help with recovery, speed up healing, and improve general health after gallbladder surgery.

When trying to get healthy again after surgery, it's important to have a deep understanding of nutritional needs, such as including certain nutrients and food groups to help the body heal best. A complete plan for nutrition after surgery includes important things like meeting nutritional needs, getting enough fiber for healthy digestion, staying hydrated, and making sure that macronutrients are distributed evenly.

Needs for Nutrition After Surgery

After treatment of the gallbladder, the body needs a lot of different nutrients to help repair tissues and keep the metabolism going.

Getting enough protein is important for treating wounds and muscles. After surgery, you should eat protein-rich foods like lean meats, chicken, fish, eggs, dairy products, legumes, and tofu to help your body heal and keep your immune system strong.

Adding vitamins and minerals is also important for improving general health and speeding up the healing process. Fresh fruits and veggies are great places to get phytonutrients, antioxidants, and important vitamins that can help the body's defenses, reduce inflammation, and speed up recovery. Whole grains are also a good source of complex carbs, fiber, and important nutrients that help keep your energy up and your digestive system healthy.

Caloric needs can be different for each person based on their age, gender, weight, amount of activity, and the extent of their surgery. It is very important to talk to a doctor or a trained dietitian to find out your specific nutritional needs and set healthy calorie goals to help you recover and avoid becoming malnourished.

Adding fiber to your diet for better digestive health

Eating enough fiber is very important for keeping your digestive system healthy and easing stomach pain after surgery. Some people may have temporary digestive problems after having their gallbladder removed, like diarrhea or constipation. Eating foods that are high in fiber can help control bowel movements and avoid digestive problems.

Fibre helps keep you regular by giving stools more bulk, making it easier for them to move through the digestive system, and keeping you from getting constipated. Soluble fiber, which can be found in oats, legumes, fruits, and veggies, can also help absorb extra bile acids. This lowers the risk of diarrhea and makes stools more stable.

But it's important to slowly add fiber to your diet after surgery so that you don't make your stomach problems worse.

Start with fiber-rich foods that are easy for your body to digest, like cooked veggies, fruits without the skin, and whole grains.

Then, slowly increase the amount of fiber you eat as your body can handle it. Pay attention to how much fiber each person can handle and change their fibre diet as needed to avoid pain and improve digestive health.

How Important It Is to Hydrate

Keeping yourself hydrated is important for many body processes, such as digestion, nutrient absorption, circulation, and getting rid of toxins. Making sure you stay hydrated is especially important after gallbladder surgery since being dehydrated can make stomach problems worse and slow down the healing process.

While water is the best drink for staying hydrated, herbal teas, clear broths, and reduced fruit juices can also help you meet your daily fluid needs. Aim to drink at least eight glasses of water every day, or more if your doctor tells you to stay hydrated and help your body heal properly.

Keeping an eye on the color of your pee can also be a useful way to tell if you are properly hydrated. If your urine is clear to pale yellow, it means you're drinking enough water. If your urine is dark yellow or amber, it could mean you're dehydrated and need to drink more water.

Getting the right amounts of protein, carbs, and fats

A balanced intake of macronutrients, which are protein, carbohydrates, and fats, is important for supporting many bodily processes and improving health and well-being after surgery. Every macronutrient has a specific job to do in the body and helps with different parts of repair and recovery.

Protein is an important part of the diet after surgery because it helps fix tissues, heal wounds, and keep muscles strong. To meet your higher protein needs during the recovery time, try to eat high-quality protein sources at every meal.

These can be lean meats, poultry, fish, eggs, dairy products, legumes, and tofu.

That's because carbohydrates are the body's main source of energy and are needed to power cellular processes and keep you active.

Complex carbohydrates, like those found in whole grains, fruits, vegetables, and beans, give you energy that lasts and important nutrients while keeping your blood sugar levels from rising too quickly.

Healthy fats are important for many bodily processes, such as making hormones, absorbing nutrients, and controlling inflammation. Avocados, nuts, seeds, olive oil, and fatty fish are all good sources of unsaturated fats that can help your heart health, lower inflammation, and improve your general health.

Try to get the right number of macronutrients by eating a range of foods that are high in nutrients at meals and snacks. Pay attention to portion amounts and dietary proportions to make sure you get enough nutrients and keep your caloric balance. Talking to a registered dietitian can give you advice and suggestions that are specific to your needs and tastes.

 starting a healing diet after gallbladder surgery means knowing and following some basic nutritional rules that will help you recover, improve your digestive health, and make you healthier in the long run. By focusing on nutrient-dense foods, adding fiber for digestive support, staying hydrated, and balancing macronutrients, people can speed up the healing process, reduce complications after surgery, and improve their general health and vitality.

CHAPTER 3
MAKING A MEAL PLAN THAT WILL NOURISH YOU

After surgery on the gallbladder, it's important to follow a carefully planned and nutritious meal plan to help the body heal and recover as quickly as possible. People who have had surgery on their gallbladder should use this complete guide to help them make a rehab meal plan that will help them heal. This guide aims to give you useful information on how to handle your diet after surgery for long-term health by including healing recipes, meal plans, and expert advice.

Making a meal plan for your recovery:

Making a meal plan for healing after gallbladder surgery requires careful thought about many things, such as the person's dietary needs, the stage of recovery, and their nutritional needs.

The main goal of the meal plan is to help the body heal, ease stomach pain, and slowly add foods that help the digestive system work. At first, you should focus on eating foods that are easy for your body to break down, like lean proteins, cooked veggies, whole grains, and healthy fats.

It's important to stay away from foods that are spicy, high in fat, or hard to digest because they can make symptoms worse and slow down healing. While making a meal plan, it can be helpful to talk to a doctor or a registered dietitian about your specific needs and tastes.

How to Get More Done with Meal Prepping:
Effective meal planning can speed up the healing process after surgery and make sure that healthy meals are always available. When you're cooking, try to use a variety of nutrient-dense foods and keep amounts small so you don't overeat or put

too much stress on your digestive system. To keep track of how fresh your meals are, use meal prep methods like cooking in bulk, dividing them into smaller containers, and writing the date on them.

Instead of frying or using too much oil, cook your food by steaming, boiling, or baking, which are all good for your stomach. To make food preparation easier and cooking time shorter, think about adding pre-cut fruits and vegetables, precooked grains, and lean proteins. Making plans ahead of time and having food on hand can help people make sure they eat a healthy, balanced diet while they are recovering.

Examples of meal plans for different stages of recovery:

People who have had gallbladder surgery can use sample meal plans to help them through the different stages of their healing. As soon as possible after surgery, you should focus on eating foods that are easy to digest to keep your stomach pain to a minimum and help your body heal. As an example, breakfast could be muesli with mashed bananas, lunch could be steamed veggies with grilled chicken and dinner could be baked fish with quinoa.

As you get better and your digestive system starts to work better, slowly start eating foods like whole grains, beans, and healthy fats that you had to avoid before. In the later stages of recovery, lunch might be a quinoa salad with mixed veggies and avocado, and dinner might be roasted sweet potatoes with salmon. It's important to pay attention to what your body is telling you and make changes to your meal plan based on your tastes and tolerances.

After gallbladder surgery, you can help your body heal and stay healthy for a long time by following a well-balanced meal plan that is tailored to your stage of recovery.

CHAPTER 4
HOW TO COOK TO GET BETTER

After treatment of the gallbladder, it's important to cook in ways that make food easier to digest and put less stress on the digestive system. Steaming is one of the best ways to cook because it keeps the nutrition in the food and makes it easier to digest. Steamed veggies, fish, and chicken are all great choices because they are easy on the stomach and give you the nutrients you need to get better. Boiling is another good way to cook, especially for grains and veggies. Vegetables can be easier to stomach if you boil them until they are soft. This helps the fibres get broken down.

Popping grains like rice or quinoa in water can also help soften them, which makes them easier on the stomach. These ways of cooking make sure that the body gets the nutrients it needs without putting extra stress on the digestive system. This helps the body heal more quickly.

During the recovery time, it's important to put digestive health first, but that doesn't mean giving up flavor. Many tasty seasoning ideas won't hurt your gut health but will make food taste better.

You could use fresh plants and spices, like mint, ginger, and turmeric, which not only make the food taste better but also help the digestive system. Ginger is especially good for soothing the stomach and getting rid of nausea, which makes it a great choice for food after surgery. Adding citrus drinks like lime or lemon can also make food taste better without adding extra fat or calories. Aromatic foods like garlic and onions can also be added to give the food more depth of flavor without making most people miserable. You can make tasty meals that help your body heal from surgery and please your taste buds by experimenting with different herbs, spices, and aromatics.

While you're healing from gallbladder surgery, it's important to make changes to recipes that are good for you and your health. One way is to focus on eating foods that are easy to digest and don't hurt the stomach, like whole grains, lean proteins, and cooked veggies.

For instance, replacing fried foods with cooked or grilled ones can help you eat less fat and feel better in your stomach. Also, eating smaller meals more often can help keep your gut system from getting too full and help your body absorb nutrients better.

Another thing to think about is adding fiber-rich foods like fruits, vegetables, and legumes to your diet. These can help avoid constipation, which is a common problem after surgery. Adding healthy fats from foods like nuts, seeds, and eggs can also improve your health and make it easier for your body to absorb nutrients. By carefully changing recipes, you can make meals that are both comfortable and healthy while you're recovering, which will help you heal faster and stay healthy in the long run.

CHAPTER 5
SUPERFOODS THAT HEAL

When you are starting to get better after surgery on your gallbladder, you must pay close attention to what you eat. It's amazing how much the foods you eat can affect your healing process, making it go faster and less painful. This detailed guide goes into great detail about the idea of healing superfoods and how they can be used in meals for people who have recently had surgery. These superfoods are full of important minerals, vitamins, and nutrients that help the body heal, lower inflammation, and boost immunity. All of these things are necessary for a full recovery.

Adding Ingredients That Reduce Inflammation

When the body is hurt or traumatized, including during surgery, it naturally reacts with inflammation. However, too much inflammation can make the healing process take longer and cause pain.

Adding anti-inflammatory foods to your diet after surgery can help reduce swelling and speed up the healing process. It is known that foods high in omega-3 fatty acids, like walnuts, and flaxseeds, and fatty fish like salmon and sardines, can help reduce inflammation. These foods can help reduce pain and swelling, which will make your healing go more smoothly overall. Spices like turmeric and ginger can also help you heal because they have strong anti-inflammatory properties and are easy to add to many recipes.

Using nutrient-dense foods to boost your immune system

Keeping your immune system strong is important for quick healing after gallbladder surgery. Eating foods that are high in nutrients is an important part of healing because it helps your immune system and general health. Adding a range of fruits and veggies to your diet gives your body the vitamins, minerals, and antioxidants it needs to stay healthy. Citrus foods, like oranges, grapefruits, and lemons, have a lot of vitamin C, which is known to help the immune system. Foods that are dark and leafy, like spinach, kale, and Swiss chard, are full of folate and vitamins A, C, and K. These vitamins help the immune system work and fix tissues. Adding foods that are high in vitamin E, like bananas, nuts, and seeds, can also boost your immune system and help you heal after surgery.

if you want to fully recover from gallbladder surgery, you need to eat a lot of healing vitamins. By eating foods that are high in nutrients and low in inflammation, you can speed up the mending process, ease pain, and support your long-term health. It's important to put your diet first if you want to recover well from surgery, whether you're using healing recipes, meal plans, or professional advice.

CHAPTER 6
COLLECTION OF RECIPES FOR HEALING AND TASTEFUL FOODS

It is very important to stick to a planned recovery diet after gallbladder surgery to help the body heal and avoid problems. This complete guide is meant to help you figure out the best way to eat after surgery. It includes meal plans, healing recipes, and health advice from experts for long-term success. Focusing on healthy foods and getting a wide range of nutrients can help you get better and improve your health in general.

Breakfast treats to get you off to a good start

Eating a healthy breakfast first thing in the morning is important for getting your energy back and helping your body heal after gallbladder surgery. Choose foods that are easy for your body to break down and are good for you while still giving you the nutrients you need.

Adding lean meats, healthy fats, and fiber-rich carbs to your breakfast can help keep your blood sugar levels steady and make you feel full all morning.

Smoothies made with Greek yogurt, veggies, berries, and flaxseeds are a great way to start the day. This blend is full of healthy nutrients that will help your healing. It has protein, vitamins, minerals, and antioxidants. For a warm and filling breakfast instead, try a bowl of muesli with sliced bananas, almonds, and honey drizzled on top.

Eggs are another great breakfast food because they are full of healthy nutrients like choline and vitamin D and high in high-quality protein.

Making scrambled eggs with sautéed veggies is a good idea. For extra fiber, serve an omelet with vegetables and whole-grain toast.

Adding whole-grain cereals, low-fat dairy products, and fresh veggies to your breakfast routine can also help mix up your morning meals and give you the nutrients you need for a quick recovery.

Try out different flavor mixes and combinations to find breakfast treats that you like and that meet your dietary needs.

Healthy Soups and Stews

Soups and stews are warm and healthy foods that can help your digestive system feel better and keep you hydrated after gallbladder surgery. To get the most nutritional value out of them, choose homemade versions made with fresh ingredients and little added salt.

Make your chicken or veggie broth to use as the base for your soups and stews. By simmering bones or veggie scraps with water, herbs, and spices, you can make a tasty and nutrient-dense broth that can be used as the base for many recipes.

To help your muscles heal and fix, add protein-rich foods like beans, lentils, lean meats, and poultry to your soups and stews. Eat a range of veggies, like leafy greens, carrots, celery, and onions, to get more fiber and keep your digestive system healthy.

Whole grains like brown rice, quinoa, or barley can be added to soups and stews to make them more filling and healthier. These healthy foods give you complex carbs and important nutrients like magnesium, selenium, and B vitamins that help your body make energy and stay healthy.

If you want to improve the taste and smell of your soups and stews, try adding different herbs, spices, and aromatics, like garlic, ginger, turmeric, and fresh herbs. When choosing ingredients and seasonings, keep in mind your own dietary needs and tastes.

Healthy Sides and Salads

Salads and side foods are flexible choices that can go with any meal and give you the nutrients and water you need.

Mix different kinds of fresh fruits, veggies, whole grains, and lean proteins to make salads and sides that are good for you and will help you heal after gallbladder surgery.

Start by making a colorful salad with spinach, kale, arugula, and other leafy greens. Add chopped veggies like tomatoes, cucumbers, bell peppers, and carrots on top of the salad. To feel fuller and help your muscles heal, add protein-rich foods like grilled chicken, salmon, tofu, or beans.

As you make salads and sides, try adding things like nuts, seeds, dried fruits, and cheese to try out different textures and tastes. Whole grains like quinoa, bulgur, and farro can be added to help digestion and your health in general. They contain fiber and complex carbohydrates that are good for you.

Heart-healthy oils like olive oil or avocado oil can be used to make your dressings. Add vinegar, orange juice, herbs, and spices for extra flavor and health benefits.

Watch your serving sizes and don't add too many high-calorie items like cheese, croutons, and creamy dressings.

You can add healthy side foods like roasted vegetables, steamed greens, whole-grain pilafs, or bean salads to your meals to make them more complete and help your body absorb more nutrients. Try to use a range of colors, textures, and tastes to make meals that are balanced and satisfying and that will help you on your recovery path.

Main Courses That Warm You Up

Main foods are the most important parts of your meals because they give you the energy and nutrients that you need to heal from gallbladder surgery.

Pick foods that are comforting and healthy, easy to digest, and gentle on your digestive system. These foods should also fill your hunger and taste preferences.

To help your muscles heal and fix, choose lean protein sources like chicken, fish, tofu, or beans and peas. To keep the natural flavors and textures of your foods while cutting down on added fats and oils, try cooking them in ways like baking, grilling, steaming, or poaching.

Adding different colored veggies to your main dishes, like broccoli, cauliflower, zucchini, squash, and bell peppers, will help your digestive health and increase the amount of fiber you eat. Try cooking your food in different ways, like baking, sautéing, or stir-frying, to make the taste and texture better.

For a healthy base for your main meals, make whole grains like brown rice, quinoa, couscous, or whole-wheat pasta. These complex carbohydrates give you long-lasting energy and important nutrients like fiber, vitamins, and minerals that are good for your health.

Use herbs, spices, marinades, and sauces made with natural ingredients like garlic, ginger, lemon, and herbs to make your main dishes taste better.

When choosing ingredients and spices to meet your needs, keep in mind any food restrictions or preferences you may have.

Soft snacks and desserts

As part of a healthy diet after surgery, desserts and snacks can be enjoyed in moderation. They can help you feel satisfied and enjoy your healing. To keep your blood sugar stable and improve your health as a whole, choose healthy foods that are low in added sugars and refined starches.

For a change of pace, try fruit-based treats like grilled peaches, baked apples, or mixed berry compote. Serve with Greek yogurt or nuts for extra flavour and texture. These naturally sweet treats are good for you because they are full of vitamins, minerals, and antioxidants that help your body heal.

You could make your own snacks like energy balls, granola bars, or trail mix with healthy things like nuts, seeds, dried fruits, and whole grains.

These snacks are easy to carry around and give you the energy and nutrients you need to get through the day.

Treat yourself to treats like dark chocolate bars, air-popped popcorn, or small amounts of your favorite dessert every once in a while, to satisfy your cravings and keep you from feeling deprived.

As part of a healthy diet after surgery, watch how much of these treats you eat and enjoy them in moderation.

Pay attention to your body's signals for hunger and fullness and savour each bite when you eat desserts and snacks. This is an example of thoughtful and intuitive eating.

Think about how different foods affect your body and mind, and choose foods that are good for your general health.

Additionally, for the best healing after gallbladder surgery, it is important to stick to a structured diet that includes healthy foods, staying hydrated, and mindful eating. You can speed up the healing process, avoid complications, and improve your health in the long run by using healing recipes, meal plans, and expert advice in your daily life.

Try out different tastes, textures, and cooking methods to make meals that are both enjoyable and healthy, and that fit your specific dietary needs and tastes. To make sure you get better and stay healthy in the future, remember to pay attention to your body, take care of yourself, and talk to a doctor or nurse if you need to.

CHAPTER 7
<u>IMPORTANT DIETARY THOUGHTS</u>

It is very important to follow a special diet after having gallbladder surgery to heal properly and be healthy generally. People may have problems with their diets, though, because they have food intolerances, allergies, or special dietary needs like being a vegetarian or vegan. This complete guide to the best diet after surgery will talk about how to handle these special food issues properly, giving you useful information, tips, and expert advice to make sure your recovery goes smoothly.

How to Deal with Food Allergies and Intolerances: People who have had surgery on their gallbladder often have changes in their digestive system that make them sensitive to or unable to handle certain foods. Having bloating, gas, diarrhea, or other stomach problems can be a sign of these intolerances.

To effectively deal with food intolerances, you need to find the foods that make your symptoms worse and remove them from your diet. Keeping a food log can help you figure out what foods are making your symptoms worse and track them after meals. As soon as you know what foods set off your symptoms, you should focus on eating more lean proteins, cooked veggies, fruits, and whole grains. Taking digestive aids like probiotics, digestive enzymes, and fiber pills may also help with digestive problems and improve gut health while you're healing.

People with food allergies need to stay away from allergenic foods that can cause bad effects. Peanuts, tree nuts, shrimp, dairy, eggs, soy, and wheat are all common foods that can cause allergies. To avoid accidentally being exposed to allergens, read food labels carefully and ask about ingredients when you eat out.

To make sure meals are safe and enjoyable, replace allergenic ingredients in recipes with safe options. Talking to a trained dietitian or allergist can help you navigate food allergies and create a healthy, allergen-free diet that meets your entire nutritional needs.

Making changes to recipes to meet specific dietary needs:

People who have had gallbladder surgery need to change meals so that they can meet their specific dietary needs. This is especially important if they have food intolerances, allergies, or a vegetarian or vegan lifestyle. Many recipes can be changed to fit different dietary needs without affecting the taste or nutritional value, as long as you are creative and clever. For example, you can use healthier ingredients like olive oil, coconut milk, or plant-based cheese instead of butter, cream, and cheese in standard recipes that call for those things.

When changing recipes, keep these things in mind:

1. To meet the protein needs of vegetarian or vegan meals, swap out animal-based proteins for plant-based ones like tofu, tempeh, legumes, and quinoa.

2. To help people who are sensitive to gluten or have celiac disease, try making with gluten-free flour like chickpea flour, coconut flour, or almond flour.

3. Use a range of herbs, spices, and citrus flavors to make food taste better without adding too much salt, sugar, or fat which is bad for you.

4. Choose cooking ways that don't add a lot of fat, like baking, steaming, grilling, or sautéing with little oil.

5. Watch your portions and don't eat too much. Big meals can stress out your digestive system and make your pain after surgery worse.

By thinking about and creatively changing recipes, people can enjoy a varied and enjoyable diet that helps them reach their recovery goals and meets their specific dietary needs.

For people on vegetarian or vegan diets, getting better after gallbladder surgery can be harder because they can't eat the high-fat animal goods that are usually part of regular meals. But if you plan and pay attention to what your body needs, veggie, and vegan options can be both tasty and good for you while you're healing. To help you eat more plant-based foods after surgery, here are some tips:

1. To help your body heal and rebuild muscles, eat lots of plant-based protein sources like nuts, seeds, tofu, lentils, edamame, tofu, and tempeh.

2. As part of your meals, eat a range of colorful fruits and veggies to get the vitamins, minerals,

antioxidants, and fiber your body needs for good digestion and immune health.

3. To help your body absorb fat-soluble vitamins and feel full, eat healthy fats in moderation from foods like avocados, olive oil, nuts, and seeds.

4. If you want to replace dairy products in recipes without changing the taste or texture, try almond milk, coconut yogurt, cashew cheese, and nutritional yeast.

5. Focus on eating whole foods that have been processed as little as possible. Eat fewer highly processed veggies or vegan convenience foods, which may be high in added sugars, sodium, and fats that are bad for you.

You might also want to talk to a registered dietitian who specializes in vegetarian and vegan nutrition to make sure that the foods you eat will help you recover and stay healthy in the long run.

They can give you personalised advice, help you plan your meals, and suggest supplements you might need to make up for any possible nutrient deficits.

Overall, people who are healing from gallbladder surgery need to make sure they take care of any special dietary needs they may have, like food intolerances, allergies, or personal food preferences. People can enjoy a varied and enjoyable diet after surgery that helps them heal, supports digestive health, and improves their long-term health by figuring out what foods cause their symptoms, coming up with new ways to cook old favorites, and making smart food choices.

CHAPTER 8
LIFESTYLE ADVICE FOR THE BEST RECOVERY

After treatment of the gallbladder, recovery is a very important time when the body needs special care and support to heal properly. In addition to medical help, changes in living are very important for this recovery process. Using lifestyle tips that are designed to help the body heal faster can greatly improve the general outcome of surgery. Here, we talk about why exercise is important after surgery, how to deal with stress in a way that helps you heal, and how to make a supportive setting for recovery.

Why exercise is important after surgery:

After gallbladder surgery, physical exercise is very important for the healing process. Even though it's important to give the body enough rest right after the operation, slowly adding light exercises and movements is helpful for many reasons.

For starters, being active can help avoid problems like blood clots and muscle loss that can happen from being immobile for a long time. Doing light workouts also improves blood flow, which makes it easier for oxygen and nutrients to get to tissues and speeds up the healing process. However, it's important to talk to a medical professional to figure out the right level of exercise based on your recovery progress and any specific limitations.

How to Deal with Stress to Get Better:

Stress can slow down the body's ability to heal after surgery. Using effective stress management methods is therefore necessary for promoting the best recovery. Meditation, deep breathing exercises, and progressive muscle relaxation are all mind-body techniques that can help lower stress and improve your overall health and well-being. Along with helping to ease stress and anxiety, these methods also boost the immune system, which speeds up the healing process. Doing fun things, practicing awareness, and reaching out to others for support can also help you deal with stress better and feel better emotionally while you're recovering.

Setting up a supportive setting that is good for recovery is very important for a quick and easy recovery after gallbladder surgery. This includes a lot of different things, like physical comfort, mental support, and practical help.

It is very important to have a comfortable and restful place to live, with enough room for rest, food, and easy access to basic amenities. Building a network of family, friends, and healthcare workers who can help you can also be very helpful for emotional support and motivation during your recovery. Talking to loved ones about your needs and limitations in a clear way can help you get the help and understanding you need.

In addition, getting help with daily chores and responsibilities can reduce stress and make it easier to focus on recovery.

People who are having surgery on their gallbladder can improve their chances of healing and long-term health by creating a supportive atmosphere.

people who are having gallbladder surgery should follow lifestyle tips that will help them heal as quickly as possible. People can speed up the healing process and improve their long-term health by understanding how important exercise is, using effective stress management methods, and making their environment supportive.

Working with medical experts, using social support networks, and putting yourself first are all important parts of a complete plan for recovery after surgery. People can get through the recovery process with strength, confidence, and, in the end, better health if they carefully follow these lifestyle rules.

CHAPTER 9
QUESTIONS PEOPLE ASK OFTEN

Worries People Have About Diets and Recovery

Patients who have had surgery on their liver often have a lot of questions about what they can eat and how to heal. One of their main worries is how to change what they eat to help them heal and get better as quickly as possible. People need to understand these worries and healthily deal with them during the time after surgery.

Answers from experts to frequently asked questions

It's important to give expert answers to frequently asked questions (FAQs) about food and recovery after gallbladder surgery so that you can ease people's worries. These answers must come from medical professionals and are specifically made to help people get better. By giving patients full answers to these questions, healthcare workers can give patients the power to make smart choices and start eating in ways that help them heal.

Nutritional Things to Think About After Surgery on the Gallbladder

After having surgery on their gallbladder, people need to be very careful about what they eat to help them heal and avoid problems. Since not having a gallbladder changes how fats are digested and absorbed, food changes are needed to reduce pain and improve health in general. To get better faster after surgery, patients should focus on eating a balanced diet full of important nutrients while also being aware of any dietary limits.

Taking Care of Digestive Issues

After gallbladder surgery, a lot of people have digestive problems like gas, bloating, and diarrhea. This is mostly because of changes in bile flow and fat absorption. Diet changes are very important for getting rid of these symptoms. People who are sick are told to eat foods that are easy for their bodies to digest, like fruits, veggies, lean proteins, and whole grains.

 Also, it's important to limit the amount of high-fat and greasy foods you eat because they can make stomach problems worse. By slowly reintroducing certain foods and keeping a food log, you can find your triggers and make the diet fit your needs.

Focusing on Hydration

Staying hydrated is important for your health in general and your healing after surgery.

Getting enough fluids can help avoid problems like dehydration, speed up the healing process, and keep your digestive system working well.

Patients should try to drink a lot of water throughout the day and not too much coffee or sugary drinks.

Drinks that are high in electrolytes, herbal teas, and clear broths can also help you reach your water goals.

Keeping an eye on your pee color and frequency can help you figure out how well you're drinking. Pale yellow urine is best.

Adding Nutritional and Healing Foods

Some nutrients and foods have healing qualities that can help you get better after gallbladder surgery. Anti-inflammatory foods, like fatty fish, leafy veggies, and berries, can help reduce swelling and speed up the healing process. Adding omega-3 fatty acid-rich foods to your diet, like flaxseeds, walnuts, and salmon, can also help your heart health and lower inflammation. Foods that are high in probiotics, like yogurt, kefir, and fermented veggies, can help keep your gut healthy and make digestion easier. This can help with digestive problems that many people have after surgery.

Tips for Planning Meals for the Best Recovery

Meal planning is important to make sure that people follow their surgeon's advice about what to eat after surgery and have the best possible recovery.

Patients should plan their meals so that they include a range of nutrient-dense foods and pay attention to how much they eat and how often they eat. Meals should be well-balanced, with lots of fruits and veggies, healthy fats, complex carbs, and lean proteins. Batch cooking and meal prepping can speed up the process of making meals, which can help people stick to their diet while they are recovering. Also, getting help from a trained dietitian can help you make meal plans that are specific to your nutritional needs and tastes.

Dealing with Social and Emotional Problems

People who have had gallbladder surgery may have trouble with their social and emotional lives as they adjust to changes in their food and deal with physical pain. It is important to handle these worries and help patients as they go through their recovery process.

Support groups, open communication with healthcare providers, and getting help from mental health professionals can all help surgery patients deal with the emotional effects of their procedure and keep a positive view of their recovery.

Having family and friends help plan and prepare meals can also create a supportive environment and make it easier for patients to follow dietary advice.

After gallbladder surgery, the priority is to get better as quickly as possible. However, following long-term dietary guidelines is important for keeping the gallbladder healthy and your general health in good shape.

Patients are told to eat lots of fruits, veggies, whole grains, and fiber and not too many processed foods, saturated fats, or refined sugars. Getting regular exercise, controlling your weight, and learning how to relax are all important parts of a healthy lifestyle that is good for your gallbladder.

Patients can lower their chance of gallstones and improve their digestive health and wellness over time by making these habits a part of their daily lives.

 addressing common concerns about diet and recovery after gallbladder surgery needs a complete approach that includes long-term dietary guidelines, managing symptoms, staying hydrated, healing foods, meal planning strategies, and social and emotional support.

Medical professionals can help patients get better and stay healthy in the long run by giving them expert answers to frequently asked questions and giving them information and tools to help them on their way. Key factors in helping patients follow dietary advice and improving outcomes after surgery are clear communication, personalised direction, and ongoing support.

CONCLUSION

Understanding the ideas behind the gallbladder surgery recovery diet is important for a speedy recovery and long-term health. People can speed up their recovery, control their digestive symptoms, and enjoy a better quality of life after surgery by following dietary rules, eating healing foods, and making changes to their lifestyle.

Healthcare workers, registered dietitians, and other experts can help with specific needs and concerns during the recovery process by giving personalised advice and support. People who have had gallbladder surgery can face the challenges of recovery with confidence and strength if they have the right information and tools. In the end, they will have better health results and a higher quality of life.

www.ingramcontent.com/pod-product-compliance
Lightning Source LLC
Chambersburg PA
CBHW060807260726
48660CB00002B/820